THE SMOKING EPIDEM

Counting the cost in
Northern Ireland

THE
SMOKING EPIDEMIC

Counting the cost in
Northern Ireland

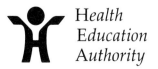

Health
Education
Authority

Report compiled by
Ken Johnson, Consultant Statistician
Christine Callum, Statistician, HEA
Amanda Killoran, Head of Health Policy, HEA

© Health Education Authority 1991
ISBN 1 85448 375 7

Health Education Authority
Hamilton House
Mabledon Place
London WC1H 9TX

Typesetting by Chapterhouse, Formby
Printed in Great Britain

Contents

Acknowledgements   vi

Foreword   vii

Introduction   1

Section 1   Trends in smoking prevalence in the UK   3

Section 2   Deaths attributable to smoking in the UK   5

Section 3   Life expectancy of smokers compared with non-smokers   9

Section 4   NHS hospital costs of diseases attributable to smoking   11

Section 5   Geographical distribution of deaths, hospital admissions, and costs: Northern Ireland   12

Appendices   1. The estimation of smoking-attributable deaths   45

  2. Life-table analysis   49

  3. Deaths by geographical area   51

  4. Hospital admissions and expenditures   52

References   54

Acknowledgements

We are grateful for the expert advice and comments given by Sir Richard Doll, Richard Peto and Nicholas Wald, and for the support of Nigel Smith, the former manager of the HEA's Smoking Education Programme, whose initiative this was, and Katie Aston for her excellent co-ordination role as project officer.

We would also like to thank Mersey Regional Health Authority for assistance with data processing, and the DoH, OPCS, the Health Intelligence Unit of the Welsh Health Common Services Agency, The Regional Information Branch of DHSS Northern Ireland, and the Registrar General's Office, Northern Ireland for providing the mortality and NHS data. We also thank the American Cancer Society for permission to use data from the Cancer Prevention Study II to estimate smokers' relative mortality risks.

This publication was produced in collaboration with the Welsh Health Promotion Authority, the Health Promotion Agency for Northern Ireland, the Health Education Board for Scotland, ASH (England), ASH (Northern Ireland) and ASH (Scotland), and the British Medical Association.

We also acknowledge the predecessors of this publication: *The Big Kill: Smoking Epidemic in England and Wales*, *The Scottish Epidemic* and *Smoking: Disease and Death in Northern Ireland*.

Foreword

Smoking is the single largest preventable cause of death in Northern Ireland.

A total of around 2,500 people are killed by tobacco use in the province every year, and each of these premature deaths from tobacco is a tragedy for both smokers and their families and friends.

Claiming one out of every six lives, tobacco is killing more people than road traffic accidents, suicides, the 'troubles', illegal drug use and AIDS combined.

Over £17 million is spent on hospital care in the province for people who smoke, and immense costs are borne by industry, with approximately 1 million lost working days each year.

These financial costs do not adequately represent the scale of human suffering.

Thousands of people endure chronic lung conditions, heart disease and many sorts of cancers.

Through parental smoking, children are born underweight and face an increase in childhood diseases.

Despite the size of the tragedy, too few people seem to be taking the issue seriously. But major efforts are being made – and the need for them to continue is clearly illustrated in the pages of this report.

Education for young people needs greater investment; the power and influence of advertising and sponsorship needs to be challenged, and we need to ensure that in our workplaces, enclosed public places and transport facilities people are not forced to breathe other people's smoke. The human and financial costs of smoking are unparalleled.

Smoking is the single largest preventable cause of death in Northern Ireland.

Action is urgently needed to stop this unnecessary suffering.

Dr Jane Wilde MB MSc FFPHM
Executive Director
The Health Promotion Agency
for Northern Ireland

Michael A Wood MBE MIHE MIPR MRSH
Director
Ulster Cancer Foundation
(Action on Smoking and Health N. Ireland)

Introduction

The aims of *The Smoking Epidemic* are:

- to indicate the significant burden caused by smoking in the UK;
- to present the toll of deaths from smoking throughout the UK and in geographical areas within the UK;
- to identify the NHS hospital activity relating to diseases attributable to smoking, and the associated financial cost.

In 1985 the Ulster Cancer Foundation on behalf of Action on Smoking and Health (NI) published a report, 'Smoking: Disease and Death in Northern Ireland'[1]. This showed, for the first time, how the smoking epidemic affected each Health and Social Services Board, local council area, and parliamentary constituency.

This new publication shows the picture six years on. Our estimate of the number of smoking-attributable deaths reflects the advance of scientific and medical knowledge since 1985, and draws primarily on the US Surgeon General's report *Reducing the health consequences of smoking – 25 years of progress.*[2] Data for 1988 are used to describe the burden of deaths and to define hospital use and associated financial costs to the NHS related to smoking. The estimate of the number of smoking-attributable deaths takes account of reduced levels of smoking in the adult population, but it includes a number of diseases not reflected in previous estimates, and also the consequences for former smokers as well as for current smokers.

The total number of premature deaths in 1988 in the UK from smoking-attributable diseases is estimated to be approximately 111 000 (one every five minutes). This means that one in every six

1

deaths are due to smoking. There are about 2500 deaths each year in Northern Ireland alone due to smoking.

Complementary reports (14) are available for England, Wales and Scotland.

Each report has five sections:

- Section 1 describes recent trends in smoking prevalence.
- Section 2 defines the range of diseases attributable to smoking, and the number of deaths for each disease in the UK attributable to smoking is calculated.
- Section 3 compares life expectancy of smokers and non-smokers.
- Section 4 describes the hospital activity and costs relating to smoking-attributable diseases.
- Section 5 presents the burden of smoking for Northern Ireland. Tables show number of deaths, hospital admissions, and financial costs of hospital activity for each Health and Social Services Board and council area.

The appendices provide technical details relating to sources of data, definitions, and methods.

Section 1

Trends in smoking prevalence in the UK

Figure 1.1 shows recent trends in cigarette-smoking in the UK (1972–88).* In 1988, 33 per cent of men and 30 per cent of women aged 16 and over were cigarette-smokers, compared with 52 per cent of men and 41 per cent of women in 1972. Although overall levels of smoking have declined, the rate of decline has slowed during the 1980s.[7]

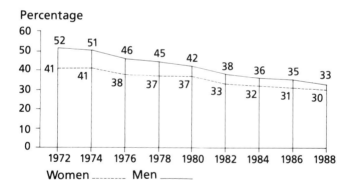

Figure 1.1. Prevalence of cigarette-smoking in adults 16 and over in the UK by sex, 1972–88.

Source: Office of Population Censuses and Surveys

---

*It is assumed that UK prevalence is the same as that for Great Britain.

3

Section 2

Deaths attributable to smoking in the UK

In recent decades an increasing number of diseases have been shown to be attributable to smoking. It is now recognised that, in addition to coronary heart disease (CHD), lung cancer, and chronic obstructive pulmonary disease (chronic bronchitis and emphysema), cigarette-smoking is a cause of cerebrovascular disease (stroke), atherosclerotic peripheral vascular disease, and cancers of the oral cavity, larynx, and oesophagus. It is thought to be a probable cause of peptic ulcer, and has been shown to be a contributory factor to bladder cancer, pancreatic cancer, and renal cancer. Associations have been, or are being, established with a number of other diseases, including aortic aneurism and cancer of the cervix.

Our list of smoking-attributable diseases was compiled from the currently available evidence on smoking and health, most of which was drawn from the US Surgeon General's (USSG) 1989 report *Reducing the health consequences of smoking – 25 years of progress.*[2] The proportions of deaths from each disease, which were estimated to have been caused by smoking, were derived from relative risks of dying for current and former cigarette-smokers compared with people who had never smoked cigarettes regularly, together with the proportions who were current and former smokers. These attributable proportions were derived for women and men separately. (See appendix 1 for details of the method.)

The table in appendix 1 shows the list of diseases, and, for women and men separately, the estimated percentages of deaths from each disease or group of diseases which were attributable to

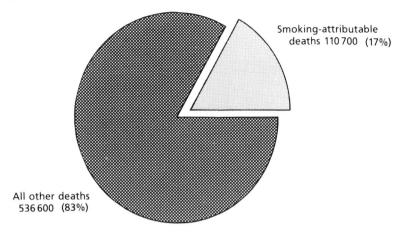

Total deaths = 647 300

Smoking-attributable
deaths 110 700 (17%)

All other deaths
536 600 (83%)

Figure 2.1. Smoking-attributable deaths as a proportion of all deaths for ages 35 and over: UK, 1988.

smoking in 1988. The number of attributable deaths for women and men together is shown in the final column of the table. They amount to nearly 110 700 deaths caused by smoking in the UK – 17 per cent of all deaths (in those 35 years and over). These proportions are shown diagramatically in Figure 2.1.

It is estimated that in 1988 in the UK:

- 32 300 lung-cancer deaths were caused by smoking – 29 per cent of all smoking-attributable deaths;
- 32 100 deaths from coronary heart disease were caused by smoking – again, 29 per cent of all smoking-attributable deaths;
- 22 000 deaths from chronic obstructive pulmonary disease (COPD) were caused by smoking – 20 per cent of all smoking-attributable deaths;
- 11 300 of deaths due to other cancers (cancers of the buccal cavity, oesophagus, larynx, bladder, kidney, pancreas and cervix) were caused by smoking – 10 per cent of all smoking-attributable deaths;

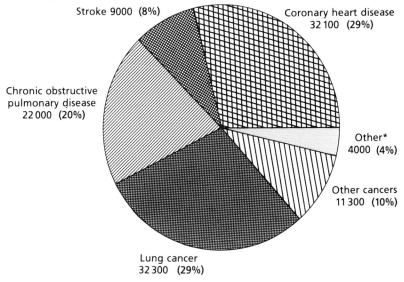

Stroke 9000 (8%)

Coronary heart disease
32 100 (29%)

Chronic obstructive
pulmonary disease
22 000 (20%)

Other*
4000 (4%)

Other cancers
11 300 (10%)

Lung cancer
32 300 (29%)

*Other = aortic aneurism and atherosclerotic peripheral vascular disease and ulcer
( ) = percentage of total deaths attributable to smoking.

Figure 2.2. Deaths attributable to smoking by disease: UK, 1988.

- 9000 deaths from stroke were caused by smoking – 8 per cent of all smoking-attributable deaths;
- 2900 deaths from aortic aneurism and atherosclerotic peripheral disease were caused by smoking – 3 per cent of all smoking-attributable deaths;
- 1000 deaths from peptic ulcer were caused by smoking – 1 per cent of all smoking-attributable deaths.

Figure 2.3, depicts the deaths attributable to smoking in relation to the total deaths from each disease, illustrating how the same number of smoking-attributable lung-cancer and CHD deaths accounts for a vastly different proportion of all deaths from the disease – respectively 81 per cent and 18 per cent.

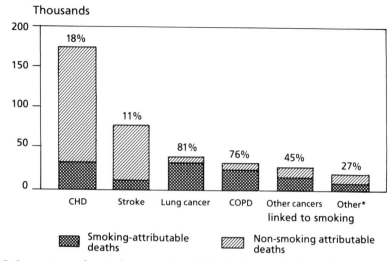

Thousands

N.B. Percentage refers to the proportion of deaths from each disease that are smoking-attributable

*Other = aortic aneurism and atherosclerotic peripheral vascular disease and ulcer.

Figure 2.3. Total deaths and deaths attributable to smoking by disease: UK, 1988.

These estimates do not include other health consequences identified in the USSG report, such as deaths due to passive smoking and impact of smoking on maternal and infant health and in this respect our total may be regarded as an understatement of the impact of smoking.

Section 3

Life expectancy of smokers compared with non-smokers

Life expectancies at different ages for cigarette-smokers and those who have never smoked cigarettes regularly are presented separately for men and women in Table 3.1. The life expectancy at a given age is the number of additional years a person can expect to live. (See appendix 2 for method and life-table proportions.)

Women aged 35 years who have never smoked regularly can expect to live a further 47 years, to the age of 82. Those who smoke regularly may expect to live a further 42 years, to the age of 77. A 35-year-old woman who smokes can thus expect to live five years fewer than a non-smoker.

Table 3.1. Life expectancy (number of years) at a given age

Men			Women		
Age	Smokers	Non-smokers	Age	Smokers	Non-smokers
35	36.5	43.5	35	41.8	46.6
40	31.7	38.8	40	37.0	41.8
45	27.1	34.1	45	32.3	37.0
50	22.7	29.4	50	27.8	32.4
55	18.7	25.0	55	23.4	27.8
60	15.0	20.8	60	19.4	23.5
65	12.0	16.9	65	15.9	19.4
70	9.3	13.5	70	12.7	15.5
75	7.2	10.7	75	10.1	12.1

For men the effect is even greater: men aged 35 years who have never been smokers may expect to live a further 44 years, to the

Table 3.2. Percentages surviving from age 35 years

Men			Women		
Age	Smokers	Non-smokers	Age	Smokers	Non-smokers
35	100	100	35	100	100
40	99	99	40	100	100
45	98	99	45	99	99
50	96	97	50	97	98
55	91	96	55	95	97
60	84	92	60	90	94
65	73	87	65	83	90
70	59	78	70	73	85
75	41	65	75	59	75

age of 79 years, while cigarette-smokers may expect to live only 37 more years, to the age of 72 years. A 35-year-old man who smokes can expect to live seven years less than a non-smoker. This means that smokers lose on average more than one day of life every week.

Table 3.2 shows, by age, the proportions surviving of those from 35 years for smokers and non-smokers (assuming they are subject to the current mortality rates). Seventeen per cent of women aged 35 years who smoke regularly will die before age 65 years, compared with 10 per cent of those who have never smoked. By age 75 years, 41 per cent of smokers will have died, compared with 25 per cent of never-smokers.

Again the effect is even more striking for men: 27 per cent of men aged 35 years who smoke cigarettes will die before age 65 years – compared with 13 per cent (more than twice the figure) for those who have never been smokers. By age 75 years, 59 per cent of smokers will have died, compared with 35 per cent of non-smokers.

Section 4

NHS hospital costs of diseases attributable to smoking

Smoking-attributable diseases impose significant costs on health-care services, including general-practice services and hospital in-patient and out-patient services. Many diseases caused by smoking are chronic, with long-term consequences for social and medical treatment and support – and not only for the NHS.

It is estimated that in 1988/89 in Northern Ireland 9300 patients were admitted to NHS hospitals on account of a disease caused by smoking. Altogether they accounted for almost 132,500 days in a hospital bed at an estimated average cost of £132 per day (including 40 per cent for overheads, and at 1990/91 prices). It has been calculated that the total annual in-patient cost to the NHS of smoking-related diseases is over £17 million. (See appendix 4 for method.) In addition, there are costs of out-patient and general-practice services to consider, which are significant.

Section 5

Geographical distribution of deaths, hospital admissions, and costs: Northern Ireland

Tables showing the number of deaths, hospital admissions, and associated hospital costs attributable to smoking are presented for the following geographical areas:

● Health and Social Services Boards
● Local council areas

Table 1 shows the number of deaths in 1988 of residents of the area, by sex and by cause for all age groups.

'Other cancers' linked to smoking include cancer of the buccal cavity, oesophagus, larynx, pancreas, kidney, bladder, and cervix. 'Chronic obstructive pulmonary disease' includes conditions such as bronchitis and emphysema. 'Other smoking attributable' diseases comprise ulcer of the stomach and duodenum, aortic aneurism, and atherosclerotic peripheral vascular disease.

For local areas, the boxplot below table 1 shows the range in the proportion of deaths caused by smoking for areas in Northern Ireland. The * shows, within this range, the percentage of deaths caused by smoking in that area.

Table 2 gives estimated figures relating to treatment by the NHS of in-patients and day-cases with diseases **caused by smoking**. All figures relate to **residents** of the area. The costs of treatment for these patients are at 1990/91 prices. Costs incurred by community and family health services are not included (for example, care by general practitioner), and therefore these costs are underestimates of the total costs to the NHS due to smoking.

Northern Ireland

- In a year about 15 813 people die in Northern Ireland. Of these **2439 (15.4% or one in six) die because of their smoking**.

- An estimated **9317** residents were **admitted to an NHS hospital** because they had an illness **caused by smoking**.

- These patients used an average of **363** hospital beds every day, at an annual **cost** to the NHS of **£17.21 million**.

TABLE 1. Deaths from smoking attributable diseases

DISEASE	DEATHS CAUSED BY SMOKING			ALL DEATHS from these diseases
	Males	Females	All	
Coronary heart disease	648	229	877	4746
Cerebrovascular disease (stroke)	127	75	202	1708
Lung cancer	450	174	624	777
Other cancers linked to smoking	158	70	228	514
Chronic obstructive pulmonary disease	308	142	450	594
Other smoking attributable	44	14	58	314
Total smoking attributable	1735	704	2439	8653

TABLE 2. Hospital care for illnesses caused by smoking

DISEASE	Annual Admissions	Beds used daily	Annual Cost £'000s
Coronary heart disease	2251	71	**3355**
Cerebrovascular disease (stroke)	496	87	**3000**
Lung cancer	1333	44	**2792**
Other cancers linked to smoking	1684	50	**3219**
Chronic obstructive pulmonary disease	2825	98	**4126**
Other smoking attributable	728	14	**716**
Total smoking attributable	9317	363	**17 209**

Note: figures may not add up due to rounding.

Eastern H&SS Board

• In a year about 6962 people die in Eastern H&SS Board. Of these **1115 (16% or one in six) die because of their smoking.**

• An estimated **4102** residents were **admitted to an NHS hospital** because they had an illness **caused by smoking.**

• These patients used an average of **160** hospital beds every day, at an annual **cost** to the NHS of **£7.58 million.**

TABLE 1. Deaths from smoking attributable diseases

DISEASE	DEATHS CAUSED BY SMOKING			ALL DEATHS from these diseases
	Males	Females	All	
Coronary heart disease	260	98	358	1966
Cerebrovascular disease (stroke)	54	35	89	781
Lung cancer	236	98	334	417
Other cancers linked to smoking	71	35	106	236
Chronic obstructive pulmonary disease	130	66	196	259
Other smoking attributable	25	7	32	136
Total smoking attributable	776	339	1115	3795

The ✳ in the box shows the % of deaths caused by smoking in Eastern H&SS Board compared with the highest and lowest proportion in Northern Ireland.

Lowest ▒▒▒▒▒▒▒▒▒▒▒▒▒▒▒▒▒▒▒▒▒▒▒▒✳▒▒▒▒▒▒▒▒▒▒▒ **Highest**
12.8%   **16%**   **17.9%**

TABLE 2. Hospital care for illnesses caused by smoking

DISEASE	Annual Admissions	Beds used daily	Annual Cost £'000s
Coronary heart disease	991	31	1477
Cerebrovascular disease (stroke)	218	38	1321
Lung cancer	587	19	1229
Other cancers linked to smoking	742	22	1417
Chronic obstructive pulmonary disease	1244	43	1817
Other smoking attributable	320	6	315
Total smoking attributable	4102	160	7576

Note: figures may not add up due to rounding.

Northern H&SS Board

• In a year about 3674 people die in Northern H&SS Board. Of these **540 (14.7% or one in seven) die because of their smoking.**

• An estimated **2165** residents were **admitted to an NHS hospital** because they had an illness **caused by smoking.**

• These patients used an average of **84** hospital beds every day, at an annual **cost** to the NHS of **£3.99 million.**

TABLE 1. Deaths from smoking attributable diseases

DISEASE	DEATHS CAUSED BY SMOKING			ALL DEATHS
	Males	Females	All	from these diseases
Coronary heart disease	165	52	217	1151
Cerebrovascular disease (stroke)	33	17	50	397
Lung cancer	97	28	125	154
Other cancers linked to smoking	30	12	42	103
Chronic obstructive pulmonary disease	66	28	94	127
Other smoking attributable	9	3	12	89
Total smoking attributable	400	140	540	2021

The **∗** in the box shows the % of deaths caused by smoking in Northern H&SS Board compared with the highest and lowest proportion in Northern Ireland.

Lowest ▒▒▒▒▒▒▒▒▒▒▒▒▒▒▒▒▒▒▒▒▒ ∗ ▒▒▒▒▒▒▒▒▒▒▒▒▒▒▒▒▒ **Highest**

12.8%   **15%**   **17.9%**

TABLE 2. Hospital care for illnesses caused by smoking

DISEASE	Annual Admissions	Beds used daily	Annual Cost £'000s
Coronary heart disease	523	16	779
Cerebrovascular disease (stroke)	115	20	697
Lung cancer	310	10	648
Other cancers linked to smoking	391	12	748
Chronic obstructive pulmonary disease	656	23	959
Other smoking attributable	169	3	167
Total smoking attributable	2165	84	3998

Note: figures may not add up due to rounding.

Southern H&SS Board

• In a year about 2714 people die in Southern H&SS Board. Of these **409 (15.1% or one in seven) die because of their smoking.**

• An estimated **1599** residents were **admitted to an NHS hospital** because they had an illness **caused by smoking.**

• These patients used an average of **62** hospital beds every day, at an annual cost to the NHS of **£2.95 million.**

TABLE 1. Deaths from smoking attributable diseases

| DISEASE | DEATHS CAUSED BY SMOKING | | | ALL DEATHS |
	Males	Females	All	from these diseases
Coronary heart disease	118	43	161	868
Cerebrovascular disease (stroke)	22	13	35	289
Lung cancer	65	27	92	115
Other cancers linked to smoking	32	8	40	79
Chronic obstructive pulmonary disease	52	22	74	96
Other smoking attributable	5	2	7	50
Total smoking attributable	294	115	409	1497

The * in the box shows the % of deaths caused by smoking in Southern H&SS Board compared with the highest and lowest proportion in Northern Ireland.

Lowest ▓▓▓▓▓▓▓▓▓▓▓▓▓▓▓▓▓▓▓▓ * ▓▓▓▓▓▓▓▓▓▓▓▓▓▓ **Highest**
112.8   **15%**   **17.9%**

TABLE 2. Hospital care for illnesses caused by smoking

DISEASE	Annual Admissions	Beds used daily	Annual Cost £'000s
Coronary heart disease	386	12	576
Cerebrovascular disease (stroke)	85	15	515
Lung cancer	229	8	479
Other cancers linked to smoking	289	9	552
Chronic obstructive pulmonary disease	485	17	708
Other smoking attributable	125	2	123
Total smoking attributable	1599	62	2954

Note: figures may not add up due to rounding.

Western H&SS Board

• In a year about 2463 people die in Western H&SS Board. Of these **375 (15.2% or one in seven) die because of their smoking.**

• An estimated **1451** residents were **admitted to an NHS hospital** because they had an illness **caused by smoking.**

• These patients used an average of **57** hospital beds every day, at an annual **cost** to the NHS of **£2.68 million.**

TABLE 1. Deaths from smoking attributable diseases

DISEASE	DEATHS CAUSED BY SMOKING			ALL DEATHS from these diseases
	Males	Females	All	
Coronary heart disease	105	36	141	761
Cerebrovascular disease (stroke)	18	10	28	241
Lung cancer	52	21	73	91
Other cancers linked to smoking	25	15	40	96
Chronic obstructive pulmonary disease	60	26	86	112
Other smoking attributable	5	2	7	39
Total smoking attributable	265	110	375	1340

The ✱ in the box shows the % of deaths caused by smoking in Western H&SS Board compared with the highest and lowest proportion in Northern Ireland.

Lowest ▓▓▓▓▓▓▓▓▓▓▓▓▓▓✱▓▓▓▓▓▓▓▓▓▓▓▓▓▓▓▓ **Highest**
12.8% **15%** **17.9%**

TABLE 2. Hospital care for illnesses caused by smoking

DISEASE	Annual Admissions	Beds used daily	Annual Cost £'000s
Coronary heart disease	351	11	522
Cerebrovascular disease (stroke)	77	14	468
Lung cancer	208	7	435
Other cancers linked to smoking	262	8	501
Chronic obstructive pulmonary disease	440	15	643
Other smoking attributable	113	2	112
Total smoking attributable	1451	57	2681

Note: figures may not add up due to rounding.

Ards

- In a year about 600 people die in Ards. Of these **99 (16.5% or one in six) die because of their smoking**.

- An estimated **354** residents were **admitted to an NHS hospital** because they had an illness **caused by smoking**.

- These patients used an average of **14** hospital beds every day, at an annual **cost** to the NHS of **£0.65 million**.

TABLE 1. Deaths from smoking attributable diseases

DISEASE	DEATHS CAUSED BY SMOKING			ALL DEATHS
	Males	Females	All	from these diseases
Coronary heart disease	23	9	31	173
Cerebrovascular disease (stroke)	6	3	9	69
Lung cancer	19	6	24	30
Other cancers linked to smoking	7	3	10	23
Chronic obstructive pulmonary disease	15	7	22	29
Other smoking attributable	2	0	2	11
Total smoking attributable	72	27	99	335

The ✱ in the box shows the % of deaths caused by smoking in Ards compared with the highest and lowest proportion in Northern Ireland.

Lowest ▒▒▒▒▒▒▒▒▒▒▒▒▒▒▒▒▒▒▒▒▒▒▒✱▒▒▒▒▒ **Highest**
12.8%   **17%**   **17.9%**

TABLE 2. Hospital care for illnesses caused by smoking

DISEASE	Annual Admissions	Beds used daily	Annual Cost £'000s
Coronary heart disease	85	3	128
Cerebrovascular disease (stroke)	19	3	114
Lung cancer	51	2	106
Other cancers linked to smoking	64	2	122
Chronic obstructive pulmonary disease	107	4	156
Other smoking attributable	28	1	27
Total smoking attributable	354	14	653

Note: figures may not add up due to rounding.

Belfast

• In a year about 3625 people die in Belfast. Of these **588 (16.2% or one in six) die because of their smoking**.

• An estimated **2136** residents were **admitted to an NHS hospital** because they had an illness **caused by smoking**.

• These patients used an average of **83** hospital beds every day, at an annual **cost** to the NHS of **£3.95 million**.

TABLE 1. Deaths from smoking attributable diseases

DISEASE	DEATHS CAUSED BY SMOKING			ALL DEATHS
	Males	Females	All	from these diseases
Coronary heart disease	129	52	181	1010
Cerebrovascular disease (stroke)	24	18	42	384
Lung cancer	125	66	191	242
Other cancers linked to smoking	35	18	53	116
Chronic obstructive pulmonary disease	68	39	107	142
Other smoking attributable	10	4	14	63
Total smoking attributable	391	197	588	1957

The ✳ in the box shows the % of deaths caused by smoking in Belfast compared with the highest and lowest proportion in Northern Ireland.

Lowest	✳	Highest
12.8%	**16%**	**17.9%**

TABLE 2. Hospital care for illnesses caused by smoking

DISEASE	Annual Admissions	Beds used daily	Annual Cost £'000s
Coronary heart disease	516	16	769
Cerebrovascular disease (stroke)	114	20	688
Lung cancer	306	10	640
Other cancers linked to smoking	386	11	738
Chronic obstructive pulmonary disease	648	22	946
Other smoking attributable	167	3	164
Total smoking attributable	2136	83	3945

Note: figures may not add up due to rounding.

Castlereagh

- In a year about 621 people die in Castlereagh. Of these **103 (16.5% or one in six) die because of their smoking**.

- An estimated **366** residents were **admitted to an NHS hospital** because they had an illness **caused by smoking**.

- These patients used an average of **14** hospital beds every day, at an annual **cost** to the NHS of **£0.68 million**.

TABLE 1. Deaths from smoking attributable diseases

DISEASE	DEATHS CAUSED BY SMOKING			ALL DEATHS from these diseases
	Males	Females	All	
Coronary heart disease	22	9	31	173
Cerebrovascular disease (stroke)	5	3	8	68
Lung cancer	28	8	36	44
Other cancers linked to smoking	7	2	9	18
Chronic obstructive pulmonary disease	8	7	15	20
Other smoking attributable	3	1	4	16
Total smoking attributable	74	29	103	339

The ✱ in the box shows the % of deaths caused by smoking in Castlereagh compared with the highest and lowest proportion in Northern Ireland.

Lowest		✱	Highest
12.8%		17%	17.9%

TABLE 2. Hospital care for illnesses caused by smoking

DISEASE	Annual Admissions	Beds used daily	Annual Cost £'000s
Coronary heart disease	88	3	132
Cerebrovascular disease (stroke)	19	3	118
Lung cancer	52	2	110
Other cancers linked to smoking	66	2	127
Chronic obstructive pulmonary disease	111	4	162
Other smoking attributable	29	1	28
Total smoking attributable	366	14	675

Note: figures may not add up due to rounding.

Down

• In a year about 565 people die in Down. Of these **79 (13.9% or one in seven) die because of their smoking**.

• An estimated **26** residents were **admitted to an NHS hospital** because they had an illness **caused by smoking**.

• These patients used an average of **13** hospital beds every day, at an annual **cost** to the NHS of **£0.62 million**.

TABLE **1. Deaths from smoking attributable diseases**

| DISEASE | DEATHS CAUSED BY SMOKING | | | ALL DEATHS |
	Males	Females	All	from these diseases
Coronary heart disease	22	8	30	163
Cerebrovascular disease (stroke)	6	3	9	80
Lung cancer	15	4	19	23
Other cancers linked to smoking	2	3	5	16
Chronic obstructive pulmonary disease	8	3	11	15
Other smoking attributable	3	0	4	16
Total smoking attributable	56	22	79	313

The ***** in the box shows the % of deaths caused by smoking in Down compared with the highest and lowest proportion in Northern Ireland.

Lowest   *****   **Highest**
12.8%   **14%**   **17.9%**

TABLE **2. Hospital care for illnesses caused by smoking**

DISEASE	Annual Admissions	Beds used daily	Annual Cost £'000s
Coronary heart disease	80	3	120
Cerebrovascular disease (stroke)	18	3	107
Lung cancer	48	2	100
Other cancers linked to smoking	60	2	115
Chronic obstructive pulmonary disease	101	4	147
Other smoking attributable	26	0	25
Total smoking attributable	333	13	615

Note: figures may not add up due to rounding.

Lisburn

• In a year about 784 people die in Lisburn. Of these **123 (15.7% or one in six) die because of their smoking**.

• An estimated **462** residents were **admitted to an NHS hospital** because they had an illness **caused by smoking**.

• These patients used an average of **18** hospital beds every day, at an annual **cost** to the NHS of **£0.85 million**.

TABLE 1. Deaths from smoking attributable diseases

DISEASE	DEATHS CAUSED BY SMOKING			ALL DEATHS from these diseases
	Males	Females	All	
Coronary heart disease	32	11	42	228
Cerebrovascular disease (stroke)	6	4	10	85
Lung cancer	27	8	35	43
Other cancers linked to smoking	8	3	12	23
Chronic obstructive pulmonary disease	17	3	20	26
Other smoking attributable	4	1	5	17
Total smoking attributable	93	30	123	422

The ***** in the box shows the % of deaths caused by smoking in Lisburn compared with the highest and lowest proportion in Northern Ireland.

Lowest ▓▓▓▓▓▓▓▓▓▓▓▓▓▓▓▓▓▓▓*****▓▓▓▓▓▓▓▓▓▓ **Highest**
12.8%   **16%**   **17.9%**

TABLE 2. Hospital care for illnesses caused by smoking

DISEASE	Annual Admissions	Beds used daily	Annual Cost £'000s
Coronary heart disease	112	4	167
Cerebrovascular disease (stroke)	25	4	149
Lung cancer	66	2	139
Other cancers linked to smoking	84	2	160
Chronic obstructive pulmonary disease	140	5	205
Other smoking attributable	36	1	36
Total smoking attributable	462	18	853

Note: figures may not add up due to rounding.

North Down

- In a year about 767 people die in North Down. Of these **123 (16.1% or one in six) die because of their smoking**.
- An estimated **452** residents were **admitted to an NHS hospital** because they had an illness **caused by smoking**.
- These patients used an average of **18** hospital beds every day, at an annual **cost** to the NHS of **£0.83 million**.

TABLE 1. Deaths from smoking attributable diseases

DISEASE	DEATHS CAUSED BY SMOKING			ALL DEATHS from these diseases
	Males	Females	All	
Coronary heart disease	32	9	42	219
Cerebrovascular disease (stroke)	7	4	11	95
Lung cancer	22	6	28	35
Other cancers linked to smoking	12	6	18	40
Chronic obstructive pulmonary disease	14	7	20	27
Other smoking attributable	3	1	4	13
Total smoking attributable	90	33	123	429

The ✱ in the box shows the % of deaths caused by smoking in North Down compared with the highest and lowest proportion in Northern Ireland.

Lowest ▨▨▨▨▨▨▨▨▨▨▨▨▨▨▨▨✱▨▨▨▨▨▨▨▨▨▨▨ **Highest**

12.8%   **16%**   **17.9%**

TABLE 2. Hospital care for illnesses caused by smoking

DISEASE	Annual Admissions	Beds used daily	Annual Cost £'000s
Coronary heart disease	109	3	163
Cerebrovascular disease (stroke)	24	4	145
Lung cancer	65	2	135
Other cancers linked to smoking	82	2	156
Chronic obstructive pulmonary disease	137	5	200
Other smoking attributable	35	1	35
Total smoking attributable	452	18	834

Note: figures may not add up due to rounding.

Antrim

- In a year about 311 people die in Antrim. Of these **40 (12.8% or one in eight) die because of their smoking**.

- An estimated **183** residents were **admitted to an NHS hospital** because they had an illness **caused by smoking**.

- These patients used an average of **7** hospital beds every day, at an annual **cost** to the NHS of **£0.34 million**.

TABLE 1. Deaths from smoking attributable diseases

DISEASE	DEATHS CAUSED BY SMOKING			ALL DEATHS from these diseases
	Males	Females	All	
Coronary heart disease	12	4	16	84
Cerebrovascular disease (stroke)	4	2	5	43
Lung cancer	7	2	9	11
Other cancers linked to smoking	2	1	3	10
Chronic obstructive pulmonary disease	3	1	5	6
Other smoking attributable	1	0	2	8
Total smoking attributable	30	10	40	162

The ✶ in the box shows the % of deaths caused by smoking in Antrim compared with the highest and lowest proportion in Northern Ireland.

Lowest ▓✶▓▓▓▓▓▓▓▓▓▓▓▓▓▓▓▓▓▓▓▓▓▓▓▓▓▓▓▓▓▓▓▓▓▓▓▓▓ **Highest**
   12.8% 13%   **17.9%**

TABLE 2. Hospital care for illnesses caused by smoking

DISEASE	Annual Admissions	Beds used daily	Annual Cost £'000s
Coronary heart disease	44	1	66
Cerebrovascular disease (stroke)	10	2	59
Lung cancer	26	1	55
Other cancers linked to smoking	33	1	63
Chronic obstructive pulmonary disease	56	2	81
Other smoking attributable	14	0	14
Total smoking attributable	183	7	338

Note: figures may not add up due to rounding.

Ballymena

• In a year about 592 people die in Ballymena. Of these **87 (14.7% or one in seven) die because of their smoking**.

• An estimated **349** residents were **admitted to an NHS hospital** because they had an illness **caused by smoking**.

• These patients used an average of **14** hospital beds every day, at an annual **cost** to the NHS of **£0.64 million**.

TABLE 1. Deaths from smoking attributable diseases

DISEASE	DEATHS CAUSED BY SMOKING			ALL DEATHS from these diseases
	Males	Females	All	
Coronary heart disease	25	9	33	183
Cerebrovascular disease (stroke)	5	3	7	62
Lung cancer	16	3	20	24
Other cancers linked to smoking	4	2	5	16
Chronic obstructive pulmonary disease	14	3	18	23
Other smoking attributable	2	1	3	21
Total smoking attributable	66	21	87	329

The ***** in the box shows the % of deaths caused by smoking in Ballymena compared with the highest and lowest proportion in Northern Ireland.

Lowest	*****	Highest
12.8%	**15%**	**17.9%**

TABLE 2. Hospital care for illnesses caused by smoking

DISEASE	Annual Admissions	Beds used daily	Annual Cost £'000s
Coronary heart disease	84	3	126
Cerebrovascular disease (stroke)	19	3	112
Lung cancer	50	2	105
Other cancers linked to smoking	63	2	121
Chronic obstructive pulmonary disease	106	4	155
Other smoking attributable	27	1	27
Total smoking attributable	349	14	644

Note: figures may not add up due to rounding.

Ballymoney

- In a year about 209 people die in Ballymoney. Of these **29 (13.8% or one in seven) die because of their smoking.**

- An estimated **123** residents were **admitted to an NHS hospital** because they had an illness **caused by smoking.**

- These patients used an average of **5** hospital beds every day, at an annual **cost** to the NHS of **£0.23 million.**

TABLE 1. Deaths from smoking attributable diseases

DISEASE	DEATHS CAUSED BY SMOKING			ALL DEATHS from these diseases
	Males	Females	All	
Coronary heart disease	8	2	10	49
Cerebrovascular disease (stroke)	2	1	3	27
Lung cancer	7	0	7	8
Other cancers linked to smoking	1	2	3	8
Chronic obstructive pulmonary disease	4	1	5	7
Other smoking attributable	1	0	1	4
Total smoking attributable	23	6	29	103

The ✱ in the box shows the % of deaths caused by smoking in Ballymoney compared with the highest and lowest proportion in Northern Ireland.

Lowest	✱	Highest
12.8%	**14%**	**17.9%**

TABLE 2. Hospital care for illnesses caused by smoking

DISEASE	Annual Admissions	Beds used daily	**Annual Cost £'000s**
Coronary heart disease	30	1	**44**
Cerebrovascular disease (stroke)	7	1	**40**
Lung cancer	18	1	**37**
Other cancers linked to smoking	22	1	**42**
Chronic obstructive pulmonary disease	37	1	**55**
Other smoking attributable	10	0	**9**
Total smoking attributable	123	5	**227**

Note: figures may not add up due to rounding.

Carrickfergus

• In a year about 267 people die in Carrickfergus. Of these **48 (17.9% or one in six) die because of their smoking**.

• An estimated **157** residents were **admitted to an NHS hospital** because they had an illness **caused by smoking**.

• These patients used an average of **6** hospital beds every day, at an annual **cost** to the NHS of **£0.29 million**.

TABLE 1. Deaths from smoking attributable diseases

DISEASE	DEATHS CAUSED BY SMOKING			ALL DEATHS
	Males	Females	All	from these diseases
Coronary heart disease	11	4	15	84
Cerebrovascular disease (stroke)	2	1	3	22
Lung cancer	11	4	15	19
Other cancers linked to smoking	2	1	4	9
Chronic obstructive pulmonary disease	7	2	9	12
Other smoking attributable	1	0	1	5
Total smoking attributable	35	13	48	151

The ✱ in the box shows the % of deaths caused by smoking in Carrickfergus compared with the highest and lowest proportion in Northern Ireland.

Lowest ▓▓▓▓▓▓▓▓▓▓▓▓▓▓▓▓▓▓▓▓▓▓▓▓▓▓▓▓▓▓▓▓▓▓▓ ✱ **Highest**
12.8%   **17.9%**

TABLE 2. Hospital care for illnesses caused by smoking

DISEASE	Annual Admissions	Beds used daily	Annual Cost £'000s
Coronary heart disease	38	1	57
Cerebrovascular disease (stroke)	8	1	51
Lung cancer	23	1	47
Other cancers linked to smoking	28	1	54
Chronic obstructive pulmonary disease	48	2	69
Other smoking attributable	12	0	12
Total smoking attributable	157	6	291

Note: figures may not add up due to rounding.

Coleraine

- In a year about 544 people die in Coleraine. Of these **75 (13.7% or one in seven) die because of their smoking.**

- An estimated **321** residents were **admitted to an NHS hospital** because they had an illness **caused by smoking.**

- These patients used an average of **12** hospital beds every day, at an annual cost to the NHS of **£0.59 million.**

TABLE 1. Deaths from smoking attributable diseases

DISEASE	DEATHS CAUSED BY SMOKING			ALL DEATHS from these diseases
	Males	Females	All	
Coronary heart disease	27	7	34	177
Cerebrovascular disease (stroke)	4	3	7	62
Lung cancer	11	2	13	16
Other cancers linked to smoking	6	2	7	14
Chronic obstructive pulmonary disease	7	5	13	17
Other smoking attributable	0	0	1	9
Total smoking attributable	55	20	75	295

The ★ in the box shows the % of deaths caused by smoking in Coleraine compared with the highest and lowest proportion in Northern Ireland.

Lowest	★	Highest
12.8%	14%	17.9%

TABLE 2. Hospital care for illnesses caused by smoking

DISEASE	Annual Admissions	Beds used daily	Annual Cost £'000s
Coronary heart disease	77	2	116
Cerebrovascular disease (stroke)	17	3	103
Lung cancer	46	2	96
Other cancers linked to smoking	58	2	111
Chronic obstructive pulmonary disease	97	3	142
Other smoking attributable	25	0	25
Total smoking attributable	321	12	592

Note: figures may not add up due to rounding.

29

Cookstown

- In a year about 299 people die in Cookstown. Of these **46 (15.3% or one in seven) die because of their smoking**.

- An estimated **176** residents were **admitted to an NHS hospital** because they had an illness **caused by smoking**.

- These patients used an average of **7** hospital beds every day, at an annual **cost** to the NHS of **£0.33 million**.

TABLE 1. Deaths from smoking attributable diseases

DISEASE	DEATHS CAUSED BY SMOKING			ALL DEATHS
	Males	Females	All	from these diseases
Coronary heart disease	16	5	21	113
Cerebrovascular disease (stroke)	3	1	4	28
Lung cancer	8	1	9	11
Other cancers linked to smoking	2	0	3	6
Chronic obstructive pulmonary disease	4	5	9	12
Other smoking attributable	0	0	1	5
Total smoking attributable	33	13	46	175

The ★ in the box shows the % of deaths caused by smoking in Cookstown compared with the highest and lowest proportion in Northern Ireland.

Lowest	★	Highest
12.8%	**15%**	**17.9%**

TABLE 2. Hospital care for illnesses caused by smoking

DISEASE	Annual Admissions	Beds used daily	Annual Cost £'000s
Coronary heart disease	43	1	63
Cerebrovascular disease (stroke)	9	2	57
Lung cancer	25	1	52
Other cancers linked to smoking	32	1	61
Chronic obstructive pulmonary disease	53	2	78
Other smoking attributable	14	0	14
Total smoking attributable	176	7	325

Note: figures may not add up due to rounding.

30

Larne

• In a year about 303 people die in Larne. Of these **41 (13.6% or one in seven) die because of their smoking.**

• An estimated **179** residents were **admitted to an NHS hospital** because they had an illness **caused by smoking**.

• These patients used an average of **7** hospital beds every day, at an annual **cost** to the NHS of **£0.33 million.**

TABLE 1. Deaths from smoking attributable diseases

DISEASE	DEATHS CAUSED BY SMOKING			ALL DEATHS from these diseases
	Males	Females	All	
Coronary heart disease	12	6	17	99
Cerebrovascular disease (stroke)	2	1	4	33
Lung cancer	5	5	10	13
Other cancers linked to smoking	2	1	3	8
Chronic obstructive pulmonary disease	4	2	6	8
Other smoking attributable	1	1	1	9
Total smoking attributable	26	15	41	170

The **✱** in the box shows the % of deaths caused by smoking in Larne compared with the highest and lowest proportion in Northern Ireland.

Lowest ▓▓▓▓▓▓▓▓✱▓▓▓▓▓▓▓▓▓▓▓▓▓▓▓▓▓▓▓▓▓▓▓▓▓▓ **Highest**

12.8%   **14%**   **17.9%**

TABLE 2. Hospital care for illnesses caused by smoking

DISEASE	Annual Admissions	Beds used daily	Annual Cost £'000s
Coronary heart disease	43	1	64
Cerebrovascular disease (stroke)	9	2	57
Lung cancer	26	1	53
Other cancers linked to smoking	32	1	62
Chronic obstructive pulmonary disease	54	2	79
Other smoking attributable	14	0	14
Total smoking attributable	179	7	330

Note: figures may not add up due to rounding.

Magherafelt

- In a year about 293 people die in Magherafelt. Of these **47 (15.9% or one in six) die because of their smoking**.
- An estimated **173** residents were **admitted to an NHS hospital** because they had an illness **caused by smoking**.
- These patients used an average of **7** hospital beds every day, at an annual **cost** to the NHS of **£0.32 million**.

TABLE 1. Deaths from smoking attributable diseases

DISEASE	DEATHS CAUSED BY SMOKING			ALL DEATHS from these diseases
	Males	Females	All	
Coronary heart disease	15	3	18	90
Cerebrovascular disease (stroke)	3	1	4	34
Lung cancer	5	3	8	10
Other cancers linked to smoking	3	1	4	9
Chronic obstructive pulmonary disease	9	2	11	14
Other smoking attributable	2	0	2	10
Total smoking attributable	36	11	47	167

The * in the box shows the % of deaths caused by smoking in Magherafelt compared with the highest and lowest proportion in Northern Ireland.

Lowest ·· * ······················ **Highest**
12.8%   **16%**   **17.9%**

TABLE 2. Hospital care for illnesses caused by smoking

DISEASE	Annual Admissions	Beds used daily	Annual Cost £'000s
Coronary heart disease	42	1	63
Cerebrovascular disease (stroke)	9	2	56
Lung cancer	25	1	52
Other cancers linked to smoking	31	1	60
Chronic obstructive pulmonary disease	52	2	76
Other smoking attributable	13	0	14
Total smoking attributable	173	7	319

Note: figures may not add up due to rounding.

Moyle

• In a year about 160 people die in Moyle. Of these **21 (13.3% or one in eight) die because of their smoking.**

• An estimated **94** residents were **admitted to an NHS hospital** because they had an illness **caused by smoking.**

• These patients used an average of **4** hospital beds every day, at an annual cost to the NHS of **£0.17 million**.

TABLE 1. Deaths from smoking attributable diseases

DISEASE	DEATHS CAUSED BY SMOKING			ALL DEATHS from these diseases
	Males	Females	All	
Coronary heart disease	8	2	10	51
Cerebrovascular disease (stroke)	3	1	3	24
Lung cancer	2	1	2	3
Other cancers linked to smoking	0	0	0	1
Chronic obstructive pulmonary disease	4	1	5	6
Other smoking attributable	0	0	1	8
Total smoking attributable	17	4	21	93

The ★ in the box shows the % of deaths caused by smoking in Moyle compared with the highest and lowest proportion in Northern Ireland.

Lowest ▓▓▓✸▓▓ **Highest**
12.8% 13%   **17.9%**

TABLE 2. Hospital care for illnesses caused by smoking

DISEASE	Annual Admissions	Beds used daily	Annual Cost £'000s
Coronary heart disease	23	1	**34**
Cerebrovascular disease (stroke)	5	1	**30**
Lung cancer	13	0	**28**
Other cancers linked to smoking	17	1	**33**
Chronic obstructive pulmonary disease	29	1	**41**
Other smoking attributable	7	0	**8**
Total smoking attributable	94	4	**174**

Note: figures may not add up due to rounding.

Newtownabbey

• In a year about 696 people die in Newtownabbey. Of these **109 (15.7% or one in six) die because of their smoking**.

• An estimated **410** residents were **admitted to an NHS hospital** because they had an illness **caused by smoking**.

• These patients used an average of **16** hospital beds every day, at an annual **cost** to the NHS of **£0.76 million**.

TABLE 1. Deaths from smoking attributable diseases

DISEASE	DEATHS CAUSED BY SMOKING			ALL DEATHS from these diseases
	Males	Females	All	
Coronary heart disease	31	10	41	221
Cerebrovascular disease (stroke)	5	3	7	62
Lung cancer	25	7	32	39
Other cancers linked to smoking	8	2	10	22
Chronic obstructive pulmonary disease	10	6	17	22
Other smoking attributable	1	1	3	10
Total smoking attributable	80	30	109	376

The ✶ in the box shows the % of deaths caused by smoking in Newtownabbey compared with the highest and lowest proportion in Northern Ireland.

Lowest ▨▨▨▨▨▨▨▨▨▨▨▨▨▨▨▨▨✶▨▨▨▨▨▨▨ **Highest**
12.8%   **16%**   **17.9%**

TABLE 2. Hospital care for illnesses caused by smoking

DISEASE	Annual Admissions	Beds used daily	Annual Cost £'000s
Coronary heart disease	99	3	148
Cerebrovascular disease (stroke)	22	4	132
Lung cancer	59	2	123
Other cancers linked to smoking	74	2	142
Chronic obstructive pulmonary disease	124	4	182
Other smoking attributable	32	1	31
Total smoking attributable	410	16	757

Note: figures may not add up due to rounding.

Armagh

• In a year about 530 people die in Armagh. Of these **87 (16.5% or one in six) die because of their smoking**.

• An estimated **312** residents were **admitted to an NHS hospital** because they had an illness **caused by smoking**.

• These patients used an average of **12** hospital beds every day, at an annual **cost** to the NHS of **£0.58 million**.

TABLE 1. Deaths from smoking attributable diseases

DISEASE	DEATHS CAUSED BY SMOKING			ALL DEATHS from these diseases
	Males	Females	All	
Coronary heart disease	26	8	34	178
Cerebrovascular disease (stroke)	4	3	6	57
Lung cancer	18	6	24	30
Other cancers linked to smoking	5	2	7	16
Chronic obstructive pulmonary disease	10	5	14	19
Other smoking attributable	1	0	2	12
Total smoking attributable	64	24	87	312

The ✱ in the box shows the % of deaths caused by smoking in Armagh compared with the highest and lowest proportion in Northern Ireland.

Lowest	✱	**Highest**
12.8%	**17%**	**17.9%**

TABLE 2. Hospital care for illnesses caused by smoking

DISEASE	Annual Admissions	Beds used daily	Annual Cost £'000s
Coronary heart disease	75	2	112
Cerebrovascular disease (stroke)	17	3	101
Lung cancer	45	1	94
Other cancers linked to smoking	56	2	108
Chronic obstructive pulmonary disease	95	3	139
Other smoking attributable	24	0	24
Total smoking attributable	312	12	577

Note: figures may not add up due to rounding.

LOCAL COUNCIL AREA
Banbridge

• In a year about 294 people die in Banbridge. Of these **43 (14.7% or one in seven) die because of their smoking.**

• An estimated **173** residents were **admitted to an NHS hospital** because they had an illness **caused by smoking.**

• These patients used an average of **7** hospital beds every day, at an annual **cost** to the NHS of **£0.32 million.**

TABLE 1. Deaths from smoking attributable diseases

DISEASE	DEATHS CAUSED BY SMOKING			ALL DEATHS from these diseases
	Males	Females	All	
Coronary heart disease	15	5	20	108
Cerebrovascular disease (stroke)	4	1	5	35
Lung cancer	5	2	7	9
Other cancers linked to smoking	2	1	3	6
Chronic obstructive pulmonary disease	6	2	8	10
Other smoking attributable	0	0	1	5
Total smoking attributable	32	12	43	173

The **✱** in the box shows the % of deaths caused by smoking in Banbridge compared with the highest and lowest proportion in Northern Ireland.

Lowest ▬▬▬▬▬▬▬▬▬▬▬✱▬▬▬▬▬▬▬▬▬▬▬ **Highest**
12.8%   **15%**   **17.9%**

TABLE 2. Hospital care for illnesses caused by smoking

DISEASE	Annual Admissions	Beds used daily	Annual Cost £'000s
Coronary heart disease	42	1	63
Cerebrovascular disease (stroke)	9	2	56
Lung cancer	25	1	52
Other cancers linked to smoking	31	1	60
Chronic obstructive pulmonary disease	53	2	77
Other smoking attributable	14	0	14
Total smoking attributable	173	7	320

Note: figures may not add up due to rounding.

36

Craigavon

- In a year about 700 people die in Craigavon. Of these **99 (14.1% or one in seven) die because of their smoking**.

- An estimated **412** residents were **admitted to an NHS hospital** because they had an illness **caused by smoking**.

- These patients used an average of **16** hospital beds every day, at an annual **cost** to the NHS of **£0.76 million**.

TABLE 1. Deaths from smoking attributable diseases

DISEASE	DEATHS CAUSED BY SMOKING			ALL DEATHS
	Males	Females	All	from these diseases
Coronary heart disease	27	12	**38**	216
Cerebrovascular disease (stroke)	4	3	**7**	64
Lung cancer	17	8	**25**	31
Other cancers linked to smoking	10	2	**12**	22
Chronic obstructive pulmonary disease	10	5	**14**	19
Other smoking attributable	2	1	**2**	9
Total smoking attributable	69	30	**99**	361

The ✴ in the box shows the % of deaths caused by smoking in Craigavon compared with the highest and lowest proportion in Northern Ireland.

Lowest	✴	Highest
12.8%	14%	17.9%

TABLE 2. Hospital care for illnesses caused by smoking

DISEASE	Annual Admissions	Beds used daily	**Annual Cost £'000s**
Coronary heart disease	100	3	**149**
Cerebrovascular disease (stroke)	22	4	**133**
Lung cancer	59	2	**123**
Other cancers linked to smoking	75	2	**143**
Chronic obstructive pulmonary disease	125	4	**183**
Other smoking attributable	32	1	**32**
Total smoking attributable	412	16	**762**

Note: figures may not add up due to rounding.

Dungannon

- In a year about 466 people die in Dungannon. Of these **65 (13.9% or one in seven) die because of their smoking**.

- An estimated **275** residents were **admitted to an NHS hospital** because they had an illness **caused by smoking**.

- These patients used an average of **11** hospital beds every day, at an annual **cost** to the NHS of **£0.51 million**.

Table 1. Deaths from smoking attributable diseases

DISEASE	DEATHS CAUSED BY SMOKING			ALL DEATHS from these diseases
	Males	Females	All	
Coronary heart disease	21	8	29	157
Cerebrovascular disease (stroke)	4	2	5	45
Lung cancer	6	2	8	10
Other cancers linked to smoking	7	1	8	15
Chronic obstructive pulmonary disease	8	5	13	17
Other smoking attributable	2	0	2	11
Total smoking attributable	47	18	65	255

The ✱ in the box shows the % of deaths caused by smoking in Dungannon compared with the highest and lowest proportion in Northern Ireland.

Lowest	✱	Highest
12.8%	**14%**	**17.9%**

Table 2. Hospital care for illnesses caused by smoking

DISEASE	Annual Admissions	Beds used daily	Annual Cost £'000s
Coronary heart disease	66	2	99
Cerebrovascular disease (stroke)	15	3	89
Lung cancer	39	1	82
Other cancers linked to smoking	50	1	95
Chronic obstructive pulmonary disease	83	3	122
Other smoking attributable	21	0	21
Total smoking attributable	275	11	507

Note: figures may not add up due to rounding.

Newry and Mourne

• In a year about 724 people die in Newry and Mourne. Of these **111 (15.4% or one in six) die because of their smoking**.

• An estimated **427** residents were **admitted to an NHS hospital** because they had an illness **caused by smoking**.

• These patients used an average of **17** hospital beds every day, at an annual **cost** to the NHS of **£0.79 million**.

TABLE 1. Deaths from smoking attributable diseases

DISEASE	DEATHS CAUSED BY SMOKING			ALL DEATHS from these diseases
	Males	Females	All	
Coronary heart disease	29	10	39	209
Cerebrovascular disease (stroke)	6	4	10	88
Lung cancer	19	9	28	35
Other cancers linked to smoking	8	2	10	20
Chronic obstructive pulmonary disease	18	5	24	31
Other smoking attributable	0	1	1	13
Total smoking attributable	80	31	111	396

The ✱ in the box shows the % of deaths caused by smoking in Newry and Mourne compared with the highest and lowest proportion in Northern Ireland.

Lowest	✱	Highest
12.8%	**15%**	**17.9%**

TABLE 2. Hospital care for illnesses caused by smoking

DISEASE	Annual Admissions	Beds used daily	**Annual Cost £'000s**
Coronary heart disease	103	3	**154**
Cerebrovascular disease (stroke)	23	4	**138**
Lung cancer	61	2	**128**
Other cancers linked to smoking	77	2	**147**
Chronic obstructive pulmonary disease	129	4	**189**
Other smoking attributable	33	1	**33**
Total smoking attributable	427	17	**788**

Note: figures may not add up due to rounding.

Fermanagh

• In a year about 599 people die in Fermanagh. Of these **87 (14.5% or one in seven) die because of their smoking.**

• An estimated **353** residents were **admitted to an NHS hospital** because they had an illness **caused by smoking.**

• These patients used an average of **14** hospital beds every day, at an annual **cost** to the NHS of **£0.65 million.**

TABLE 1. Deaths from smoking attributable diseases

DISEASE	DEATHS CAUSED BY SMOKING			ALL DEATHS from these diseases
	Males	Females	All	
Coronary heart disease	24	8	31	168
Cerebrovascular disease (stroke)	6	3	9	72
Lung cancer	9	6	14	18
Other cancers linked to smoking	7	4	10	24
Chronic obstructive pulmonary disease	17	3	20	25
Other smoking attributable	2	1	3	11
Total smoking attributable	64	23	87	318

The ✱ in the box shows the % of deaths caused by smoking in Fermanagh compared with the highest and lowest proportion in Northern Ireland.

Lowest	✱	Highest
12.8%	15%	17.9%

TABLE 2. Hospital care for illnesses caused by smoking

DISEASE	Annual Admissions	Beds used daily	Annual Cost £'000s
Coronary heart disease	85	3	127
Cerebrovascular disease (stroke)	19	3	113
Lung cancer	51	2	106
Other cancers linked to smoking	64	2	122
Chronic obstructive pulmonary disease	107	4	156
Other smoking attributable	28	1	27
Total smoking attributable	353	14	652

Note: figures may not add up due to rounding.

Limavady

- In a year about 234 people die in Limavady. Of these **41 (17.5% or one in six) die because of their smoking**.

- An estimated **138** residents were **admitted to an NHS hospital** because they had an illness **caused by smoking**.

- These patients used an average of **5** hospital beds every day, at an annual **cost** to the NHS of **£0.25 million**.

TABLE 1. Deaths from smoking attributable diseases

DISEASE	DEATHS CAUSED BY SMOKING			ALL DEATHS from these diseases
	Males	Females	All	
Coronary heart disease	11	3	14	71
Cerebrovascular disease (stroke)	2	1	3	27
Lung cancer	12	1	13	16
Other cancers linked to smoking	4	1	5	10
Chronic obstructive pulmonary disease	2	3	4	6
Other smoking attributable	0	0	1	3
Total smoking attributable	32	9	41	133

The ✱ in the box shows the % of deaths caused by smoking in Limavady compared with the highest and lowest proportion in Northern Ireland.

Lowest   ✱ **Highest**
12.8%   **17.9%**

TABLE 2. Hospital care for illnesses caused by smoking

DISEASE	Annual Admissions	Beds used daily	Annual Cost £'000s
Coronary heart disease	33	1	50
Cerebrovascular disease (stroke)	7	1	45
Lung cancer	20	1	41
Other cancers linked to smoking	25	1	47
Chronic obstructive pulmonary disease	42	1	61
Other smoking attributable	11	0	11
Total smoking attributable	138	5	254

Note: figures may not add up due to rounding.

Derry

- In a year about 839 people die in Derry. Of these **130 (15.5% or one in six) die because of their smoking**.

- An estimated **494** residents were **admitted to an NHS hospital** because they had an illness **caused by smoking**.

- These patients used an average of **19** hospital beds every day, at an annual **cost** to the NHS of **£0.91 million**.

TABLE 1. Deaths from smoking attributable diseases

DISEASE	DEATHS CAUSED BY SMOKING			ALL DEATHS
	Males	Females	All	from these diseases
Coronary heart disease	33	13	46	257
Cerebrovascular disease (stroke)	5	4	9	79
Lung cancer	19	10	28	36
Other cancers linked to smoking	8	6	13	37
Chronic obstructive pulmonary disease	19	12	31	41
Other smoking attributable	1	1	2	12
Total smoking attributable	85	45	130	462

The ★ in the box shows the % of deaths caused by smoking in Derry compared with the highest and lowest proportion in Northern Ireland.

Lowest ▨▨▨▨▨▨▨▨▨▨▨▨▨▨▨▨▨▨▨▨★▨▨▨▨▨▨▨▨▨▨▨▨▨▨ **Highest**

12.8% **16%** **17.9%**

TABLE 2. Hospital care for illnesses caused by smoking

DISEASE	Annual Admissions	Beds used daily	Annual Cost £'000s
Coronary heart disease	119	4	178
Cerebrovascular disease (stroke)	26	5	159
Lung cancer	71	2	148
Other cancers linked to smoking	89	3	171
Chronic obstructive pulmonary disease	150	5	219
Other smoking attributable	39	1	38
Total smoking attributable	494	19	913

Note: figures may not add up due to rounding.

Omagh

- In a year about 444 people die in Omagh. Of these **70 (15.8% or one in six) die because of their smoking.**

- An estimated **262** residents were **admitted to an NHS hospital** because they had an illness **caused by smoking.**

- These patients used an average of **10** hospital beds every day, at an annual **cost** to the NHS of **£0.48 million.**

TABLE 1. Deaths from smoking attributable diseases

DISEASE	DEATHS CAUSED BY SMOKING			ALL DEATHS from these diseases
	Males	Females	All	
Coronary heart disease	19	7	26	142
Cerebrovascular disease (stroke)	3	1	4	33
Lung cancer	9	3	13	16
Other cancers linked to smoking	4	2	6	14
Chronic obstructive pulmonary disease	14	5	20	26
Other smoking attributable	1	0	1	5
Total smoking attributable	51	19	70	236

The **∗** in the box shows the % of deaths caused by smoking in Omagh compared with the highest and lowest proportion in Northern Ireland.

Lowest ∗ Highest
12.8% **16%** **17.9%**

TABLE 2. Hospital care for illnesses caused by smoking

DISEASE	Annual Admissions	Beds used daily	Annual Cost £'000s
Coronary heart disease	63	2	94
Cerebrovascular disease (stroke)	14	2	85
Lung cancer	37	1	79
Other cancers linked to smoking	47	1	90
Chronic obstructive pulmonary disease	79	3	116
Other smoking attributable	20	0	20
Total smoking attributable	262	10	484

Note: figures may not add up due to rounding.

Strabane

- In a year about 347 people die in Strabane. Of these **48 (13.7% or one in seven) die because of their smoking**.

- An estimated **204** residents were **admitted to an NHS hospital** because they had an illness **caused by smoking**.

- These patients used an average of **8** hospital beds every day, at an annual **cost** to the NHS of **£0.38 million**.

TABLE 1. Deaths from smoking attributable diseases

DISEASE	DEATHS CAUSED BY SMOKING			ALL DEATHS from these diseases
	Males	Females	**All**	
Coronary heart disease	18	5	23	123
Cerebrovascular disease (stroke)	2	1	3	30
Lung cancer	3	1	4	5
Other cancers linked to smoking	2	2	4	11
Chronic obstructive pulmonary disease	8	3	11	14
Other smoking attributable	1	0	2	8
Total smoking attributable	35	12	48	191

The ✱ in the box shows the % of deaths caused by smoking in Strabane compared with the highest and lowest proportion in Northern Ireland.

Lowest ▓▓▓▓▓▓▓▓✱▓▓▓▓▓▓▓▓▓▓▓▓▓▓▓▓▓▓▓▓▓▓▓▓▓▓▓▓▓▓▓ **Highest**

12.8%   **14%**   **17.9%**

TABLE 2. Hospital care for illnesses caused by smoking

DISEASE	Annual Admissions	Beds used daily	**Annual Cost £'000s**
Coronary heart disease	49	2	**74**
Cerebrovascular disease (stroke)	11	2	**66**
Lung cancer	29	1	**61**
Other cancers linked to smoking	37	1	**71**
Chronic obstructive pulmonary disease	62	2	**90**
Other smoking attributable	16	0	**16**
Total smoking attributable	204	8	**378**

Note: figures may not add up due to rounding.

44

Appendix 1

The estimation of smoking-attributable deaths

The list of smoking-attributable diseases was derived from two major reviews, published in recent years, of the evidence concerning tobacco smoking and health. They are the International Agency for Research on Cancer monograph on tobacco smoking[4] and the US Surgeon General's (USSG) 1989 report on the health consequences of smoking[2]. Each review categorised diseases according to their established relationship to smoking, and this was used to compile our list of diseases attributable to smoking.

The proportion of deaths attributable to smoking for each disease or group of diseases is estimated from exposure-specific relative risks and prevalence. Two exposure categories were used: current smokers and former smokers. The attributable proportions were derived, separately for women and men, from the following:

$$a = \frac{p_c(r_c - 1) + p_f(r_f - 1)}{1 + p_c(r_c - 1) + p_f(r_f - 1)}$$

where p_c and p_f are, respectively, the proportions of those aged 35 years or more who are current or former regular cigarette-smokers, and r_c and r_f are, respectively, the relative risks for current and former cigarette-smokers of dying from the disease compared with the risks for those who never were regular cigarette-smokers.

The relative risks were derived from the 1982–88 Cancer Prevention Study (CPS II). This was a large prospective epidemiological survey of women and men aged 35 years or more which was carried out between 1982 and 1988 in the United States by the American Cancer Society. The past history of cigarette-smoking of the study population and the associated relative mortality risks represented the best available approximation to contemporary UK.

Current smokers' relative risks were calculated from information on deaths and exposure in five-year age groups which were available for the first four years of the study. The data were supplied to Richard Peto for use in the WHO study of smoking deaths, and the American Cancer Society gave us permission to use the data in this study too. Relative risks were calculated as the ratios of current smokers and never-smokers' five-year age-specific mortality rates, weighted where appropriate by the UK age distribution.

Proportions by age of deaths attributable to current smoking were calculated by applying the above formula with only one exposure, namely current smokers. Attributable deaths by age were then calculated and summed over all ages to give an all-age attributable proportion for current smokers, a_c. From this an all-age relative risk for current smokers was calculated as follows:

$$r_c = \frac{a_c + p_c(1 - a_c)}{p_c(1 - a_c)}$$

where a_c is the proportion of deaths attributable to current regular cigarette-smokers.

Former smokers' relative risks for the CPS II study population aged 35 years or more were published in the USSG's 1989 report. UK age-adjusted relative risks were calculated on the very crude assumption that the ratio of UK and CPS II risks is the same for former as for current smokers.

The figures for smoking prevalence, or exposure, were obtained from the 1988 *General household survey*.[3] They were standardised to the UK age distributions. An estimated 29 per cent of women and 32 per cent of men aged 35 years or more were current cigarette-smokers, and a further 22 per cent of women and 41 per cent of men had regularly smoked cigarettes in the past.

The attributable percentages were applied to the 1988 UK deaths by disease to produce an estimate of the number of deaths attributable to smoking.[5,6,7] The list of diseases, the attributable percentages for women and men separately, and the estimated number of deaths attributable to smoking in the UK in 1988 are given in Table A1.1.

Certain attributable percentages are lower than those used hitherto – notably, for example, lung-cancer deaths: 69 per cent for women and 86 per cent for men, compared with 90 per cent or more. An alternative estimate based on the CPS II study of the number of smoking-attributable deaths can be obtained by applying the non-smokers'

Table A1.1. Estimates of percentages and numbers of deaths attributable to smoking, UK 1988

	Attributable percentage			Attributable deaths		
	Men	Women	All	Men	Women	All
Coronary heart disease	24	11	18	23 573	8536	32 109
Cerebrovascular disease (stroke)	19	7	12	5507	3492	8999
Aortic aneurism and atherosclerotic peripheral vascular disease	44	15	29	2433	472	2905
Chronic obstructive pulmonary disease	80	69	76	15 525	6463	21 988
Cancer of the lung	86	69	81	23 908	8437	32 345
Cancer of the buccal cavity, oesophagus, larynx	84	48	71	4468	1478	5946
Cancer of the bladder	45	29	40	1651	491	2142
Cancer of the kidney	49	7	32	774	71	845
Cancer of the pancreas	22	30	26	716	1065	1781
Cancer of the cervix	—	29	29	—	588	588
Ulcer of stomach & duodenum	24	20	22	517	527	1044
Total				**79 072**	**31 620**	**110 692**

47

lung-cancer mortality rates to the UK population and subtracting the numbers of 'expected' deaths from the actual number of UK deaths. This method assumes equivalence between CPS II and UK non-smokers' lung-cancer mortality rates. It gives attributable percentages of 81 for women and 92 for men, which denote an additional 3275 lung-cancer deaths attributable to smoking.

This latter estimate may well be the more accurate as the method used to obtain it is the most appropriate when there is reason to think that the rate in non-smokers is relatively constant over time, as in the case of lung cancer. It cannot, however, be applied generally to all other diseases, as the rate in non-smokers for many diseases may well be changing and, in these circumstances, the method we have used reduces the risk of overestimating the effects of smoking.

Appendix 2

Life-table analysis

The construction of separate life tables for smokers and non-smokers required the estimation of UK 1988 age-specific mortality rates for current smokers and for those who had never smoked cigarettes regularly.

Age-specific mortality rates were calculated as the sum of age-specific mortality rates from smoking-attributable diseases and age-specific mortality rates from all other diseases. The first component by definition differs between current smokers and never-smokers, while the second is assumed to be the same for each.

For each smoking-attributable disease and within each age and gender category, the mortality rate for **never-smokers** was estimated from the following:

$$m_n = \frac{m_t}{1 + p_c(r_c - 1) + p_f(r_f - 1)}$$

where m_n is the disease-specific mortality rate for never-smokers and m_t is the disease-specific mortality rate for the population, which includes never-smokers, current smokers, and former smokers, and p_c and p_f are respectively the proportions in the age group who are current and former regular cigarette-smokers, and r_c and r_f are, respectively, the age-specific relative risks for current and former smokers of dying from the disease compared with the risks for those who were never cigarette-smokers.

For age groups 35–39, 40–44, ... 55–59 years, the 35–59 year relative risk was assumed. Relative risks for former smokers by age were not available. They were estimated by making the crude assumption that the ratio between former and current smokers' relative risks within each age group was the same as the all-age ratio.

For each smoking-attributable disease and within each age and gender category, the mortality rate for **current smokers** was estimated by multiplying the never-smokers' rate by the current smokers' relative risk.

Abridged life tables were constructed from the age-specific mortality rates. They describe survivorship from age 35 years of a cohort subject to these rates.

Appendix 3

Deaths by geographical area

The number of deaths in 1988 by cause, sex, and electoral government district of residence was provided by the General Register Office for Northern Ireland. The data was further aggregated to Health and Social Service Boards.

For each cause of death and separately for males and females, the proportions of deaths due to smoking (see appendix 1) were applied to the mortality statistics assembled for each geographical area. This provided estimates of the numbers of deaths caused by smoking.

Appendix 4

Hospital admissions and expenditures

(a) Hospital admissions

The number of in-patient admissions, day cases, and occupied bed days by diagnosis was provided by DHSS, Northern Ireland from their patient database. The DHSS also provided 'bottom-line' counts of the same measures of activity. This was used to adjust the data derived from the patient database, controlling it to the correct activity level for the country.

The number of patients with illnesses caused by smoking was estimated using the same proportions for each disease as were applied to the mortality data (see appendix 1). Patients with no recorded diagnosis were attributed to 'smoking' using the overall proportion derived from those patients with known diagnosis.

(b) Hospital in-patient expenditure

A further table, obtained from OPCS, identified hospital admissions (in-patients and day cases) and bed days by specialty and diagnosis. 'Direct' treatment costs at specialty level were supplied by the Department of Health.

These sources were used to estimate a cost (per bed day) for treating each disease. The estimated disease costs were multiplied by 1.685, reflecting (i) the ratio of **total** NHS inpatient and day-case expenditure to the **direct treatment** expenditure; (ii) price changes between 1990/91; and (iii) the overall average cost per case in Northern Ireland relative to that in England. The estimated costs per bed day for the main categories of smoking-related diseases are given in the table.

Table A4.1. Estimated costs per bed day, by disease group

Disease	Cost per bed day* (£)
Coronary heart disease	130
Cerebrovascular disease (stroke)	95
Lung cancer	173
Other cancers	167
Chronic obstructive pulmonary disease	115
Other 'smoking-related' diseases	115

*Costs at 1990/91 prices, including overheads.

(c) Estimation of hospital activity and expenditure for health boards and local government districts

The analysis described above derives hospital activity and costs due to smoking for residents of Northern Ireland. In order to estimate equivalent figures for residents of local government districts and health boards, the activity and cost data was apportioned according to the proportions of **total deaths** in Northern Ireland which occurred in each local area.

References

1. *Smoking: Disease and Death in Northern Ireland.* 1985. Published for Action on Smoking and Health (NI) by the Ulster Cancer Foundation.
2. US Department of Health and Human Services. 1989. *Reducing the health consequences of smoking – 25 years of progress. A report of the Surgeon General.* US Department of Health and Human Services, Public Health Service, Centres for Diseases Control, Centre for Chronic Disease Prevention and Health Promotion, Office of Smoking and Health. DHHS Publication No. (CDC) 89-8411.
3. Office of Population Censuses and Surveys. 1990. *General household survey 1988.* HMSO.
4. International Agency for Research on Cancer. 1986. IARC Monographs on the evaluation of the carcinogenic risk of chemicals to humans, Volume 38: *Tobacco Smoking.* IARC.
5. Office of Population Censuses and Surveys. 1990. *Mortality statistics, cause, England and Wales 1988*, Series DH2, No. 15.
6. General Register Office for Scotland. 1989. *Annual report 1988.* HMSO.
7. General Register Office for Northern Ireland. 1989. *Annual report 1988.* HMSO.